THE PHONE GUIDE

HOW YOUR SMARTPHONE IS EFFECTING

YOUR HEALT

KATE .P

1

Contents

CHAPTER ONE

INTRODUCTION

Smartphones have grown commonplace in the current digital era and are essential to our everyday activities. These gadgets have completely changed the way we live and work by offering a wide range of functions, from productivity and health management to communication and enjoyment. But as cellphones have become more ingrained in our daily lives, there is a rising recognition of the possible risks they pose to our health and wellbeing.

This introduction looks at both the advantages and disadvantages of using smartphones to investigate how they are affecting our health. Smartphones present threats to one's physical and mental health as well as to social interactions, even though they are incredibly beneficial in terms of connectivity, ease, and information availability. People may promote a balanced and healthy lifestyle in the digital era and make educated decisions regarding their smartphone usage by being aware of these effects.

The pervasiveness of smartphones in contemporary culture

Unquestionably, cellphones are a pervasive fixture in modern culture, influencing almost every facet of our personal and professional lives. These portable electronics are now essential instruments for work, communication, amusement, information access, and many other uses. This is an examination of their ubiquitous impact:

Communication: By providing rapid access to calls, texts, emails, and social media platforms, smartphones completely changed communication. They promote real-time interactions and teamwork by enabling people to stay in touch with friends, family, coworkers, and clients regardless of their location.

Information Access: A few taps on a smartphone can bring up a plethora of information. Users can obtain information on almost any topic via websites, search engines, news apps, and online databases, facilitating ongoing research, learning, and knowledge exchange.

Entertainment: Smartphones are great for on-the-go entertainment centers because they offer a wide range of multimedia content, such as podcasts, e-books, streaming services, gaming apps, and music platforms. They provide consumers with mobile entertainment options so they may decompress, unwind, and enjoy their preferred media at any time, anyplace.

Productivity: The abundance of productivity tools and applications available on smartphones helps to improve productivity. Smartphones help users organize their schedules, manage activities, and cooperate with others, enhancing productivity and effectiveness in both business and personal life. These tools range from calendars and task managers to note-taking apps and document editors.

Travel and Navigation: GPS technology is built into smartphones and provides precise navigation as well as real-time traffic updates. This makes it simpler for users to plan trips, locate landmarks nearby, and navigate unfamiliar routes. Travel applications facilitate smooth travel experiences by offering information about hotels, restaurants, attractions, and airlines.

Health and Fitness: Wearable technology and a variety of apps on smartphones help users achieve their fitness and health goals. Fitness monitoring applications encourage users to lead healthier lifestyles and reach their fitness objectives by recording exercise, measuring physical activity, and offering individualized health insights.

Financial Management: Users may easily and securely manage their accounts with the use of smartphone banking apps, budgeting tools, and mobile payment solutions. Mobile banking streamlines financial processes and saves time by enabling users to check account balances, transfer money, pay bills, and deposit checks from a distance.

Social networking: Through social media apps on smartphones, users can engage in online communities and social networking by connecting with friends, exchanging updates, pictures, and videos, and taking part in events and conversations. In the digital age, social media platforms have become essential for networking, community involvement, and socializing.

Emergency Assistance: In times of need, smartphones can be users' lifelines since they provide the ability to contact emergency services, call for assistance, and communicate their location with reliable connections. Emergency alert systems and safety applications offer prompt notifications and resources in the event of accidents, natural disasters, or other emergencies.

Inclusivity and Accessibility: Smartphones are accessible to people with impairments thanks to features like voice recognition, screen readers, and assistive touch functions. These functions encourage diversity and give people of all abilities the tools they need to fully engage in digital society.

All things considered, the pervasiveness of cellphones has revolutionized the way we interact, work, socialize, and get around. Smartphones bring with them unprecedented ease and connectedness, but they also bring with them worries about privacy, security, digital addiction, and the effects of constant connectivity on mental health and general wellbeing. To maintain a positive and long-lasting connection with technology, it's critical to strike a balance between maximizing the advantages of cellphones and reducing any potential negative effects as they continue to develop and become more integrated into our daily lives.

Effects on Physical Health

There are some beneficial and bad consequences on physical health that have been brought about by the widespread usage of smartphones. An outline of how cellphones can affect physical health is provided below:

Benefits:

Health Monitoring: Wearable technology and a variety of apps on smartphones make it possible to track one's health. Users are encouraged to maintain a healthy lifestyle by being able to track their heart rate, physical activity, sleep habits, and other health data.

Fitness and Exercise: By recording exercises, establishing fitness goals, and offering feedback on progress, fitness applications and wearable technology encourage users to participate in regular physical activity. They have the power to motivate people to make healthier lifestyle choices and fit exercise into their regular schedules.

Medical Assistance: Apps for smartphones are a great way to discover doctors, make appointments, get medical information, and keep track of meds. By enabling users to consult with medical professionals remotely, telemedicine apps enhance access to healthcare, particularly for those who live in distant places or have limited mobility.

Safety and Emergency Assistance: Smartphones with capabilities like location sharing, emergency calling, and safety apps provide users a feeling of security. Users might potentially save lives by promptly notifying loved ones about their whereabouts, contacting authorities, and accessing emergency assistance during emergencies.

Adverse Impacts:

Sedentary Behavior: Using a smartphone excessively can lead to sedentary behavior, which raises the risk of obesity, cardiovascular disease, and other health issues as well as a lack of physical activity. Extended durations of sitting and screen time can be detrimental to musculoskeletal function and metabolic health.

Posture Problems: "Text neck" and "tech neck," which are frequently brought on by using smartphones excessively, are typical posture-related problems that cause headaches, strain on the spine, and pain in the neck and shoulders. Looking down at a smartphone screen all the time might cause musculoskeletal abnormalities and bad posture.

Eye Strain: Using a smartphone for extended periods of time can lead to dry eyes, discomfort, and blurred vision, especially in dimly lit areas or with small letter sizes. Smartphone screens emit blue light, which can interfere with sleep cycles and aggravate digital eye fatigue.

Accidents and Distraction: Using a smartphone while operating a vehicle, walking, or performing other tasks can be hazardous and increase the chance of an accident or injury. When using a smartphone to text or browse, one's focus is taken off of their surroundings, which increases the risk of falls, collisions, and other safety issues.

Use of cellphones right before bed might interfere with sleep cycles and reduce the quality of sleep.

CHAPTER TWO

The hormone melatonin, which controls sleep-wake cycles, is suppressed by the blue light emitted by screens, making it more difficult to fall asleep and having a detrimental effect on the quantity and quality of sleep that is obtained.

Addiction and Mental Health: Overuse of smartphones can lead to behaviors that resemble addiction, including obsessive social media checking, compulsive checking, and FOMO (fear of missing out). This may have an adverse effect on one's general mental health and well-being by raising stress, anxiety, depression, and feelings of isolation or loneliness.

Radiation Exposure: Although studies on the health effects of radiation from smartphones are still in progress, some data point to possible health risks, such as an increased risk of cancer and negative effects on reproductive health, from prolonged exposure to the radiofrequency electromagnetic fields (RF-EMFs) that smartphones emit. To completely comprehend the long-term effects of smartphone radiation on human health, more research is necessary.

While smartphones have many advantages when it comes to tracking health, promoting fitness, and providing access to medical information, overuse or inappropriate use can also have negative effects on one's physical health, such as sedentary behavior, poor posture, eye strain, accidents, disturbed sleep, addiction, and possible radiation exposure. People must value moderation and balance, be aware of how they use their smartphones, and take proactive measures to minimize any negative health impacts while optimizing the positive effects of digital technology on general wellbeing.

Effects on Mental Health

Numerous consequences, both positive and negative, on mental health have been brought about by the increasing usage of smartphones. Below is a summary of the ways in which smartphones may affect mental health:

Benefits:

Access to Supportive Resources: Smartphones give users access to online support groups, mental health hotlines, therapy apps, and meditation apps. These resources promote resilience, self-care, and coping mechanisms while providing helpful tools and support for people dealing with mental health issues.

Social Connection: Through social media sites, messaging applications, video conversations, and online communities, smartphones let people connect with each other and build interpersonal relationships. They make it possible for people to maintain relationships with friends, family, and peers, which promotes social support, a sense of community, and belonging especially during periods of loneliness or isolation.

Distraction and Relaxation: Gaming apps, streaming services, e-books, and relaxation apps are just a few of the entertainment and relaxation alternatives available on smartphones. Playing games on smartphones is a great way to relieve boredom, relax, and elevate your mood in addition to offering brief stress relief.

Mindfulness and Meditation: Apps for smartphones provide stress-reduction plans, breathing exercises, guided meditation, and mindfulness exercises that support emotional control and mental health. With the use of these applications, users can improve their self-awareness and emotional resilience, manage stress and anxiety, and develop mindfulness abilities.

Adverse Impacts:

Digital Addiction: Prolonged smartphone use can result in addictive behaviors, such as obsessive screen time, compulsive checking, and trouble putting down the gadgets. Addiction to smartphones can cause problems with day-to-day functioning, damage relationships, and exacerbate depressive, anxious, and poor self-esteem sentiments.

Social Comparison and FOMO: People who use social media on their cellphones to compare their life to carefully chosen online representations of others' experiences may experience feelings of inadequacy and social comparison. Social media FOMO (fear of missing out) can result in feelings of loneliness, envy, and discontent with one's own life.

Use of smartphones right before bed can interfere with sleep cycles and reduce the quality of one's sleep. Screen blue light suppresses melatonin production, which makes it difficult to fall asleep and has a detrimental effect on the quantity and quality of sleep that is received. Sleep difficulties have been linked to exhaustion during the day, emotional swings, and cognitive decline.

Anxiety and Stress: Feelings of overwhelm, anxiety, and stress can be exacerbated by smartphones' constant connectedness and information overload. Alerts from social media, emails, and notifications might make you feel stressed out and make you constantly on guard, which can make it harder to unwind.

Cyberbullying and Harassment: Via social media sites, messaging applications, and online forums, smartphones make cyberbullying and online harassment possible. In particular for teenagers and young people, experiencing cyberbullying can have a negative impact on mental health by causing emotions of guilt, embarrassment, despair, and social disengagement.

Reduced Cognitive Functioning and Attention Span: Prolonged smartphone use has been linked to lower productivity, cognitive overload, and attention span reduction. Constant multitasking and smartphone information consumption can impede cognitive function, memory, and concentration, making it more difficult to succeed in school and at work.

Depression and Social Isolation: Research has connected increased rates of depression, loneliness, and social isolation to excessive smartphone use and social media involvement. Overuse of screens can supplant in-person conversations and deep social ties, resulting in mental anguish and feelings of alienation and detachment.

While there are many advantages to smartphones, such as easy access to resources for mental health, social interaction, and relaxation, there are also drawbacks to excessive or inappropriate use, such as the potential for digital addiction, social comparison, anxiety, insomnia, cyberbullying, depression, and cognitive impairment. To preserve mental health in the digital era, people must prioritize self-care, set boundaries, be aware of how they use their smartphones, and ask for help when they need it.

Impacts on Social Health

The way individuals connect, communicate, and build relationships has been significantly impacted by the increasing usage of cellphones, which has had an impact on social health. An outline of how cellphones affect social health is provided below:

Benefits:

Improved Connectivity: Regardless of location, people can stay in touch with friends, family, and coworkers thanks to smartphones, which enable quick communication and connectivity. Real-time connections are made possible by social media platforms, messaging apps, and video conversations, which help to build and sustain relationships over time.

Increased Social Networks: People can interact with a variety of online communities and interest groups and increase the size of their social networks by using smartphones. By facilitating networking, connecting with like-minded people, and participating in activities and hobbies that they have in common, social media platforms and online forums help people feel more integrated into society and like they belong.

Enhanced Social Support: Smartphones make it easier for people to access social networks and resources, which enables them to ask friends, family, and online communities for emotional support, guidance, and encouragement. Social media and messaging applications provide a forum for people to express their feelings, share their experiences, and get support and understanding from others—all of which contribute to resilience and emotional well-being.

Facilitated Social Activities: Smartphones make it easy and flexible to plan parties, get-togethers, and social activities. Group chats and messaging applications facilitate communication, planning, and coordination among participants, making it simpler to arrange get-togethers, exchange updates, and work together on social events or projects.

Community Engagement: By giving users access to news, information, and resources about regional events, causes, and activities, smartphones encourage civic engagement and participation. Social media platforms inspire active citizenship and community involvement by allowing users to advocate, mobilize support, and raise awareness for social change.

Adverse Impacts:

Social Comparison: Using social media on a smartphone can amplify the tendency for people to compare themselves negatively to other people based on well constructed accounts of their lives. People may feel inadequate, envious, or have low self-esteem as a result of trying to live up to the fictitious images of happiness, success, and beauty that are perpetuated online.

Reduced Face-to-Face Interaction: People who use their smartphones excessively tend to prioritize virtual communication over in-person contacts, which can negatively impact face-to-face encounters and interpersonal relationships. The quality and depth of social relationships may be diminished by distracted or surface-level conversations brought on by constant connectivity and screen usage.

Isolation and Loneliness: It is ironic that an increased tendency toward social media involvement and smartphone use has also been associated with feelings of social isolation and loneliness. Overusing cellphones can cause significant social contacts and offline connections to be replaced, which can cause alienation, loneliness, and a sense of detachment, especially in sensitive populations like older individuals and adolescents.

Cyberbullying and Harassment: Via social media sites, messaging applications, and online forums, smartphones make cyberbullying and online harassment possible. In particular among teenagers and young adults, experiencing cyberbullying can have a negative impact on mental health, self-esteem, and social relationships. It can also cause emotions of guilt, anxiety, and social disengagement.

Addiction and Dependency: Prolonged smartphone use can result in addictive and dependency-like behaviors, such as compulsive checking, a need for continual contact, and trouble putting down digital gadgets. Addiction to smartphones can harm people's general social health and well-being by taking time away from obligations, interests, and in-person social contacts.

Although smartphones have many advantages, such as increased connectivity, broader social networks, and easier access to social support, overuse or inappropriate use can also have detrimental effects on social health, such as dependency, loneliness, cyberbullying, and social comparison in addition to decreased face-to-face interaction and face-to-face interaction. In the digital age, it's critical for people to emphasize offline contacts, set limits, be aware of how they use their smartphones, and ask for help when they need it in order to keep their wellbeing and social ties strong.

Techniques for Reducing Adverse Impacts

In order to minimize the negative impacts of excessive smartphone use, proactive measures that promote balanced and thoughtful usage while optimizing the advantages of digital technology are needed. The following are a few tactics people might use to lessen the harmful effects of smartphones:

Set Usage Limits: Define boundaries and restrictions on the use of smartphones by designating daily periods or durations for their use. To impose usage limitations and stop excessive screen time, make use of features like app timers, screen time limits, and parental controls.

Establish Smartphone-Free Zones: Set aside specific times or places, including during meals, get-togethers with family, or social trips, for the use of smartphones. In these specific areas, keep smartphones out of sight and out of reach to promote meaningful talks and face-to-face contact.

CHAPTER THREE

Practice Digital Detox: Take regular pauses to recharge and unplug from continual connectivity when using smartphones and other digital gadgets. To encourage attention and lessen dependency on screens, schedule times throughout the day—such as before bedtime, during exercise, or during relaxation—when no devices are allowed.

Put Real-Life ties First: Make an investment in fostering social ties and real-life relationships by giving in-person conversations precedence over technological contact. Make time for meaningful conversations and deeper ties with friends, family, and loved ones by setting aside time for quality time spent together away from the distractions of cellphones.

Take Part in Offline Activities: Look into pastimes, passions, and pursuits that don't entail digital screens or smartphones. Get away from digital distractions and partake in hands-on tasks, artistic endeavors, or outdoor activities that foster creativity, mindfulness, and personal fulfillment.

Practice Mindful Smartphone Usage: By engaging in mindful routines and behaviors, you can develop awareness and intentionality when using smartphones. Consider why you reached for your smartphone in the first place, pay attention to how you felt both before and after using it, and make a deliberate decision about when and how to use digital technology in a thoughtful manner.

Control Notifications and Distractions: Tailor your smartphone's notification settings to reduce interruptions and distractions during the day. When working or relaxing, turn off unneeded notifications, give priority to important alerts, and use "Do Not Disturb" or silent mode.

Establish a Tech-Free Bedtime Routine: To encourage improved sleep hygiene and lessen smartphone use at night, establish a tech-free bedtime routine. Establish a digital curfew by shutting off screens at least an hour before bed, read or practice meditation, or do other peaceful hobbies to help you fall asleep and wake up feeling refreshed.

Seek Accountability and Support: Talk to friends, family, or support groups about your plans and objectives for cutting back on smartphone use. By looking for support, finding accountability partners, or participating in online communities that promote digital well-being and thoughtful technology use, you may hold yourself responsible for keeping your promises.

Exercise Self-Reflection: Consistently consider your behaviors, routines, and well-being impacting smartphone usage. Observe how using a smartphone impacts your relationships, productivity, energy levels, and mood. Then, make any necessary adjustments to bring your smartphone use in line with your healthy living objectives and values.

By putting these tips into practice, people can develop better connections with their smartphones, lessen the harmful effects of excessive use, and encourage balance and general well-being in the digital age.

Effects on Youth and Teenagers

Parents, educators, and medical experts are becoming more concerned and interested in the effects of smartphones on kids and teenagers. While there are many advantages to cellphones for communication, education, and entertainment, there are also some significant concerns and possible negative effects associated with youth smartphone use. An summary of how cellphones affect kids and teenagers may be found here:

Benefits:

Communication: Children and teenagers may stay in touch with friends, family, and peers via text messages, calls, and social media thanks to smartphones, which also make it easier for them to be connected. This strengthens bonds with others and creates a feeling of unity and belonging.

Learning & Education: Educational apps, e-books, online lessons, and information access are just a few of the educational resources and opportunities that smartphones provide for kids and teenagers. They can help with learning outside of the classroom, improve digital literacy, and offer individualized instruction based on each student's interests and learning preferences.

Entertainment and Recreation: Through social media platforms, game apps, streaming services, and multimedia material, smartphones provide kids and teenagers entertainment and recreational opportunities. In particular, these digital encounters provide chances for fun, creativity, and relaxation during downtime or leisure.

Safety and Security: By giving kids access to safety apps, emergency calling services, and location tracking, smartphones can improve their sense of safety and security. Smartphone capabilities allow parents to keep an eye on their kids' locations, contact them in an emergency, and make sure they're safe when they're not at home.

Adverse Effects:

Screen Time and Sedentary Behavior: Children and adolescents who use smartphones excessively may experience longer periods of screen time and sedentary behavior, which lowers their levels of physical activity and raises their risk of obesity, cardiovascular disease, and other health issues. Excessive use of smartphones might also hinder play outside and in-person social interactions.

Sleep Disruption: Using a smartphone right before bed might cause sleep patterns and quality issues for kids and teenagers. Screen blue light suppresses melatonin production, which makes it difficult to fall asleep and has a detrimental effect on the quantity and quality of sleep that is received. Sleep disturbances can have an impact on academic achievement, mood regulation, and cognitive function.

Cyberbullying and Online Risks: Through social networking sites, messaging applications, and online gaming communities, smartphones expose kids and teenagers to cyberbullying, online harassment, and other digital risks. Being the target of cyberbullying can have a negative impact on one's mental health, sense of self, and interpersonal connections. It can cause feelings of social disengagement, anxiety, and depression.

Social Comparison and Digital Pressures: Children and adolescents who use social media on their cellphones may be more susceptible to social comparison and digital pressures. When young people compare themselves negatively to others online, exposure to idealized images and lifestyles on social media may exacerbate feelings of inadequacy, low self-esteem, and body image issues.

Digital Addiction and dependent: Children and adolescents who use smartphones excessively may develop dependent and addiction-like behaviors, such as compulsive checking, a need for continuous connectivity, and trouble putting down the gadgets. Addiction to smartphones can affect one's ability to operate on a daily basis, interfere with schoolwork, and harm one's social and emotional connections.

Attention & Concentration: Using a smartphone during academic or recreational activities that call for prolonged focus and mental engagement might negatively impact children's and adolescents' attention span, concentration, and cognitive performance. Over time, continuous multitasking and smartphone information overload may impair cognitive development and academic achievement.

Parent-Child Relationships: When kids and teenagers use their smartphones excessively, it can take away from their quality time with parents and other family members. This can cause arguments about screen time limits, communication problems, and disengagement from family activities. Maintaining good parent-child ties and encouraging communication and bonding require striking a balance between digital and offline encounters.

While children and teenagers might benefit greatly from cellphones in terms of communication, education, and entertainment, their excessive or inappropriate use can also have detrimental effects on social interactions, academic performance, mental health, and physical health. To support young people's general wellbeing and digital resilience, parents, educators, and caregivers must be aware of their children's smartphone usage habits, set reasonable boundaries and restrictions, and offer guidance and support for responsible and balanced technology use.

Summary

In conclusion, there are a variety of ways that cellphones can affect one's physical, emotional, and social well-being. These effects can either be beneficial or negative. Although cellphones provide never-before-seen levels of connectedness, convenience, and information access, worries regarding the possible negative effects of excessive or inappropriate use on one's health have been raised by the devices' pervasiveness in contemporary culture.

Positively, cellphones have transformed communication, learning, entertainment, and healthcare accessibility by enabling people to track their health, maintain relationships, and access information and support services. Additionally, they have promoted innovation in telemedicine, remote monitoring, and health tracking, enhancing the availability and quality of healthcare.

But using cellphones excessively can also result in a number of health problems, such as being sedentary, having trouble sleeping, straining your eyes, developing a digital addiction, feeling anxious or depressed, isolating yourself from others, and engaging in cyberbullying. Overuse of screens and continual connectedness can negatively affect one's quality of life by taking away from social interactions, exercise, and mental health.

People should emphasize offline contacts and self-care activities, set boundaries and limitations on screen time, adopt mindful technology usage habits, and seek assistance and tools for managing their digital well-being in order to lessen the detrimental impacts of cellphones on their health. In addition, stakeholders including legislators, educators, medical professionals, and tech companies contribute to the development of digital literacy, appropriate and balanced smartphone use, and surroundings that encourage healthy living in the digital age.

Individuals and communities can maximize the positive effects of digital technology while reducing any negative effects by being aware of the potential health risks associated with smartphones and taking proactive measures to mitigate them. This will ultimately lead to a more positive and balanced relationship between people and technology in the modern world.

THE END